The
A
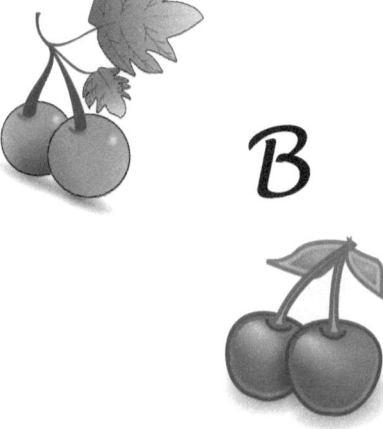
B
C's
of Nutrition

Dr. Phylis B. Canion, DCCN, FAAIM

authorHOUSE®

AuthorHouse™
1663 Liberty Drive
Bloomington, IN 47403
www.authorhouse.com
Phone: 1 (800) 839-8640

Published by AuthorHouse 10/18/2018

ISBN: 978-1-5462-6490-3 (sc)
ISBN: 978-1-5462-6489-7 (e)

Dedication

This book is dedicated to Steve, my husband and best friend since 1976. He has always been my pillar of strength and encouragement and was instrumental in my pursuit of my goals. He was there through several illnesses during our dating years and I will be forever indebted to him for his nursing skills-especially after I broke both thumbs and was unable to use either hand for six weeks. He is the BEST.

I would also like to thank my parents, my mother Emily and especially my father, Fred. He was a wonderful guinea pig in sharing my experiments, especially while learning Iridology, and Fingernail and Tongue analysis, maintaining his encouragement along the way. My sister Viv, brothers Kai and Byron and their families shared a lot of eye rolling, but now, even they have a better understanding of the roll of nutrition in our health.

A very special thank you to Dr. Dan Dugi-my friend, my mentor and the most brilliant doctor I have ever met. His encouragement, intellect and support have been an invaluable tool for which I am forever indebted. I would also like to thank Louise O'Connor and Bli Dugi for their editing skills. Without their expertise this book would have been difficult reading.

Introduction

I must begin by saying that I have a real passion for writing this book and trying to help educate individuals on the benefits and pitfalls of the food we eat daily. After living abroad for over sixteen years, and having traveled to every continent except Antarctica, I feel I have an expanded understanding of nutrition and the daily role it plays in our health and longevity. My theory: We are not only overdosing daily on food toxins, we are digging our graves with our own set of tools, our teeth.

After I earned a degree in Psychology I had a few friends that came calling to ask for help in trying to get their lives straightened out. One particular lady had a ten year old with a multitude of behavioral problems including Attention Deficit Disorder (ADD) and Attention Deficient Hyperactivity Disorder (ADHD). After several visits and no foreseen improvement, I decided to ask her one simple question that turned out to have great significance. "Does your child drink milk?" Her reply was that he drank a lot of it every day. I suggested that she remove milk from his diet for a couple of weeks and then schedule a phone consultation to further discuss the behavioral issues.

Lo' and behold, she called me back in four days, mind you-not two weeks. Her son was a different person after eliminating milk from the diet. His behavior had improved, his symptoms of allergy rhinitis (continuous runny nose) had stopped, and his constipation eased dramatically. That is when I began wondering how much of our problems, both physical and mental, were more food related than anything. With the encouragement of my husband, I began to study nutrition and earned a Diploma in Holistic Nutrition. I furthered my education by obtaining a Masters in Nutrition, becoming Board Certified as a Nutritional Consultant and earning my Doctor of Naturopathic Medicine degree.

There is more to creating and maintaining good health than exercise alone. You must first posses the mental and physical qualities that allow one's body to partake in physical activity.

I hope this simple guide will help you understand nutrition and make more educated health decisions the next time you are standing in front of instant noodles and canned sodas at the grocery market.

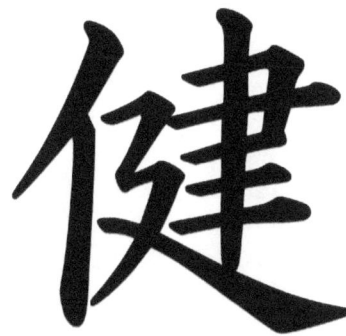 **The Japanese symbol for Health**

$\mathcal{A}$

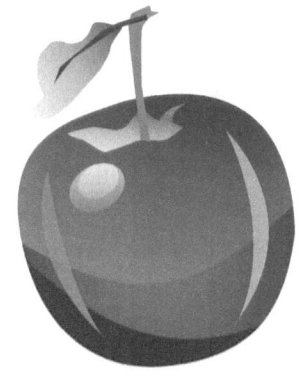

Eat at least one **apple** daily. Apples contain pectin and pectin helps pull toxins out of the body.

An **acidic** body is a disease magnet. Check your pH to be sure your system is balanced between your acid and alkaline levels. A very important factor to a healthy body is to have a balanced pH. A pH of 7 is neutral-balanced between acid and alkaline. A pH reading, below 7 is considered acidic. A pH reading above 7 is considered alkaline. pH measures the amount of hydrogen in the equilibrium condition. The acidic or alkalinity of food is measured by the pH value of the ash residue that remains after food has been metabolized by the body. The ash can be acidic, alkaline or neutral depending upon the mineral content of the food that was digested.

This is easy to determine as the common sense "bad foods" such as refined sugar, foods high in saturated fats and trans fats, meat, dairy, yeast, canned sodas, chocolate, caffeine and alcohol all leave acidic ash. Whereas, the common sense "good foods" such as salads, vegetables, fruits, etc. all leave alkaline ash.

Fact:

Vitamin A is the vitamin most likely to be deficient in the Standard American Diet.

Human Body Trivia:

At birth everyone is color blind.

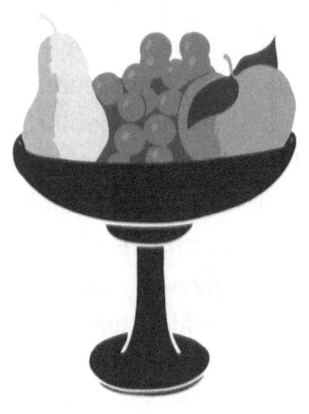

Standard **Amino Acids** serve as raw materials for the manufacture of many other cellular products, including hormones and pigments. Many amino acids act as key intermediates to aid in cellular metabolism.

Avoid **alcohol**. Alcohol impairs the transport of the amino acid trytrophan into the brain, where it is converted to serotonin to promote the natural sleep cycle.

There are three major forms of **arthritis**: osteoarthritis, rheumatoid arthritis and gout. Dietary intake has shown a strong connection to many forms of arthritis, both to cause and to cure. Societies that have a diet rich in natural foods, fiber and vegetables and low in meat, sugar, refined carbohydrates, and saturated fats, see a lower incidence of arthritis than societies that eat opposite of this approach.

Avoid **aspartame**, the artificial sweetener. Aspartame is considered an excitotoxin. Longterm damage is associated with the repeated consumption of excitatory amino acids, phenylalanine, methanol, and DKP of which there are 92 health side effects. Disorders and side effects that may be associated with aspartame

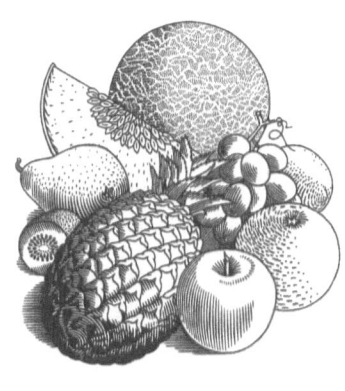

consumption include the following: poor vision, ringing in ears, neurological changes, psychological illness, shortness of breath, gastrointestinal disturbances, skin and allergy problems, and dysfunction of the endocrine and metabolic system. Aspartame toxicity may trigger, mimic or cause Chronic Fatigue Syndrome, Epstein-Barr virus, Lyme disease, Grave's disease, Meniere's disease, ALS (Lou Gehrigs disease), Epilepsy, Multiple Sclerosis, Fibromyalgia, and Attention Deficit Disorder.

Avoid consuming any products that are packaged in/or contain **Aluminum** (i.e. canned sodas, baking powder, or buffered aspirin). Aluminum blocks the action potential or electrical discharge of nerve cells, and reduces nervous system activity based on animal studies. Aluminum also inhibits important enzymes in the brain (Na-K-ATPase, and hexokinase) and may also inhibit uptake of important chemicals by nerve cells (dopamine, norepinephrine, and 5-hydroxytryptamine).

B

The **B complex** vitamins are one of the most significant groups of vitamins. As a group, they are the most easily

Fact:

Long before clinical evidence of deficiency develops, our bodies are no longer operating at peak efficiency.

Human Body Trivia:

The aorta, the largest artery in the body, is almost the diameter of a garden hose.

Breast cancer is forty times more likely to occur in women who are constipated.

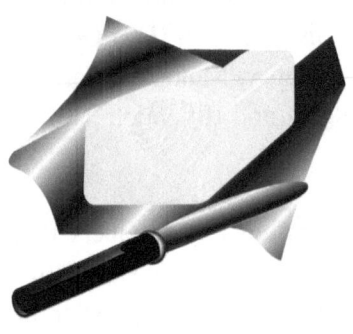

Fact:

The average American gets most of their calories from fat, with processed sugar being the second source of calories.

destroyed by cooking, improper storage, illness, stress, poor digestion and high glycemic foods. Make sure you are taking multi vitamins that contain the B Complex family: B 1- Thiamine, B 2-Riboflavin, B 3-Niacin, B-5 Panothenic Acid, B 6-Pyridoxine, B 7-Biotin, B 9-Folic Acid, and B 12-Cyanocobalamin. B vitamins are water soluble and must be replaced daily, because excess water is excreted in the urine.

Keep the **bowels** moving. Our ancestors defecated on average every 12 to 16 hours. The average time now is anywhere between 24 to 36 hours. Water and fiber play a key role in keeping our bowels flushed of toxins. If stool has ample amount of water and fiber, it will be very light tan in color.

Bones are living structures, which are forever changing. Lack of nutrients and water leaves them complaining with pain and fractures.

Butter is the king. Butter has been around for centuries and has many nutritional benefits.

C

Eliminate **caffeine** from your diet. Caffeine increases calcium loss leading to bone destruction. Long term

Food Combining Chart

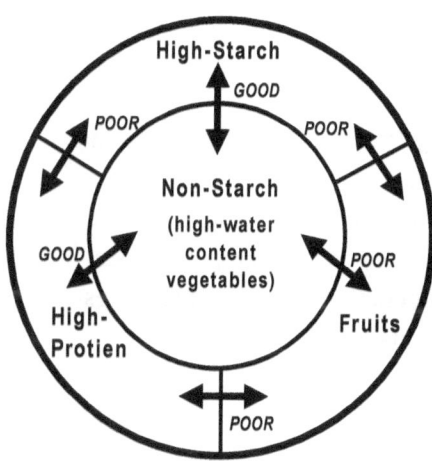

caffeine consumption effects on blood pressure has not been clearly determined, yet studies of short term effects consistently shown that consuming caffeine causes a rise in blood pressure.

Eliminate **canned sodas.** Canned sodas contribute more sugar to the Standard American Diet (SAD- coincidence of the acronym) than any other food.

Chew your food. The more you chew your food, the easier it is for the digestive juices to surround each piece in the stomach, which aids in digestion and allows nutrients to be released quicker. My suggestion; chew each mouth full at least twenty six times (when I was in England, I heard that the Queen chews each mouthful twenty five times). Not only will you be eating properly, your stomach will love you.

A **calorie** is a unit of measure for energy. Expending the amount of calories consumed daily maintains weight.

Food **combining** is dictated by digestive chemistry, which means that different foods are digested differently.

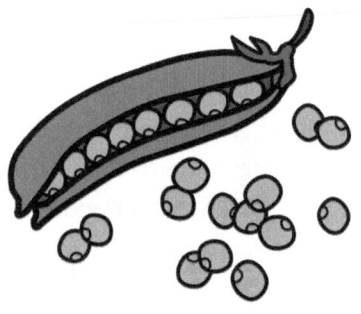

Starchy foods require an alkaline digestive medium, which is supplied initially in the mouth by the enzyme ptyalin. Protein foods require an acid medium for digestion aided by hydrochloric acid. In simpler terms-if you eat a starch with a protein, digestion is impaired or completely arrested.

The best combination is a non-starch and a high protein (i.e. broccoli and poultry or pastas and zucchini) *See chart to the left and the complete list of foods on page 41.*

The body transforms **carbohydrates** into blood sugar or glucose-the body's preferred fuel source. Most carbohydrates come from plant foods-fruits, vegetables, grains and legumes (dried beans, lentils and peas).

Cancer, composed of more than one hundred diseases, is characterized by excessive, uncontrolled growth of abnormal cells, which invade and destroy healthy tissue. Cancer is the second leading cause of death in the United States after heart disease. While cancer is not completely understood, conscious lifestyle choices can dramaticallyreduce the risk of developing cancer by sixty percent. Do not smoke, eat a healthy diet, and enjoy moderate exercise.

"The human body heals itself, and nutrition provides the resources to accomplish the task."
Hippocrates

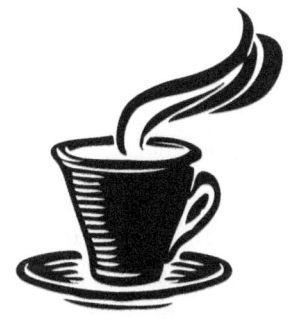

The eyes never change their size from birth, although our ears and nose never stop growing.

D

Do Not skip meals. Individuals that skip meals have a tendency to overeat during the course of a day. Even if it is just a couple of bites of something, it is always better to eat frequent small meals than eliminate meal time altogether.

Decaffeinated products are much better if they are decaffeinated naturally. Being decaffeinated naturally means that the caffeine has been removed by a water process rather than with chemicals. But remember, even decaffeinated products are not 100% decaffeinated, but 99.7% caffeine free.

The recommended **diet** is the Mediterranean Type Diet as listed on Page <u>39.</u>

Your **dose** is your poison. How much you consume daily (i.e food, drink or drugs) can be your poison.

Disease is the result of a problem and usually begins with a blockage within the system.

E

Exercise is important in helping you eliminate toxins. Not only does physical activity burn calories,

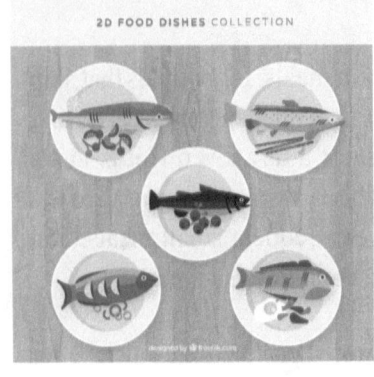

2D FOOD DISHES COLLECTION

it helps decrease appetite and should be a part of any health program.

Enzymes are the spark plugs of the body. Just like our car, our body needs everything working together to maintain a healthy environment. Enzymes are one of many specialized organic substances, composed of polymers of amino acids that act as catalysts to regulate the speed of the chemical reactions involved in the metabolism of living organisms, such as digestion.

Fruits should be consumed daily and eaten by themselves rather than in combination with other foods. When combined with other foods, the stomach will begin digesting the sweet which delays the complete digestion of the remaining food in the stomach allowing for bloating, belching and a feeling of fullness.

Fish Tips:
- Fresh fish has no smell-so a fishy smell is a sign of spoilage.
- Don't buy fish from stores that display cooked and raw fish on the same layer of ice, even if they are separated.
- Be sure that the fish is not stacked so high on the ice that it becomes heated by the light in the cooler.

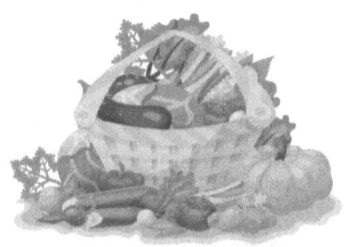

FRESH VEGETABLES

Duis aute irure dolor in reprehenderit in voluptate velit esse cillum dolore eu fugiat nulla pariatur excepteur sint occaecat cupidat.al proident, sunt in culpa qui officia deserunt mollit

Fiber is very important in our diet. Consuming at least 30-35 grams of soluble and insoluble fiber daily is what the human body requires. A high fiber diet can reduce the likelihood of hemorrhoids, appendicitis, diverticulosis and constipation. Fiber plus water can prevent constipation. Fiber increases the frequency and quantity of bowel movements, decreases the transit time of stool, decreases the absorption of toxins from the stool, and may be a preventative factor in several diseases. Fiber also decelerates the metabolism of sugar into the bloodstream.

Learn how to read **Food labels**. Food labels give you information that can help you decide what to choose as a part of an overall healthy eating plan. Not only do food labels provide you with nutrition information, they also tell you what is in a packaged food (the ingredients), whether it is organic, and contains certain health claims. The Federal Drug Administration (FDA) and the United States Department of Agriculture (USDA) regulate any health claims that companies make on their food labels. Declaring a food, *"lite", "low fat",* or *"sugar free"* (to name a few), must meet strict government definitions in order to make that claim. Foods that are labeled "USDA organic" are required to have at least 95% organic ingredients.

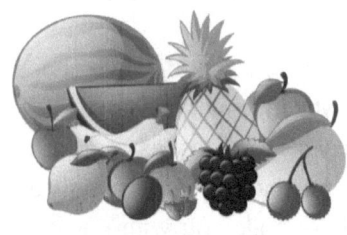

Fingernails can reflect what is happening in specific organs of the body. The thumb; reflects what is going on in the brain, and excretory system. The index finger; reflects what is happening in the liver, gall bladder and nervous system. The middle finger; indicates what is going on in the heart and circulatory system. The ring finger indicates what is going on in the reproductive organs and hormonal system. And the little finger reflects what is going on in the digestive system. An analysis will look at nail color, shape, pliability, texture and markings. A healthy system is indicated when each nail has a lunula (the little half moon) on each finger except the little finger.

Free radicals are essential compounds that are used in the body in various ways. White blood cells, which are involved in the body's defense system, use free radicals to destroy bacteria and viruses. Free radicals are also directly involved in the production of hormone like compounds called prostaglandins that help regulate many different bodily functions. The liver, which filters out toxic products from the body, uses free radicals in the process of detoxification. However, free radicals can also have a damaging effect on healthy cells in the body if they

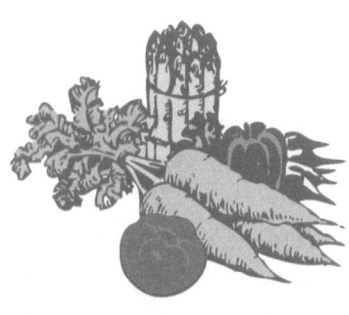

become too numerous because free radicals are chemically unstable. The body is equipped with its own natural defense system that guards against an overabundance of free radicals. It produces special free radical scavengers called antioxidants that neutralize them before vital molecules are damaged. The result: they are harmlessly absorbed into the body.

Fats, like trans fats and rancid fats, should be avoided completely. Cell membranes, nerve tissue, and steroid hormones all require healthy fats. Unhealthy fats interfere with these functions and structures.

G

Know the **glycemic** index (GI) of foods. The glycemic index is the rate at which a carbohydrate triggers a rise in circulating blood sugar. Carbohydrate foods that break down quickly during digestion have a high glycemic index, whereas carbohydrate foods that break down slowly, and release glucose more gradual into the blood, have a low glycemic value. Your body maintains a certain glucose level in order to serve the brain and the central nervous system. To maintain this availability, the body stores glucose in the muscles and in the liver.

In one square inch of our hand, we have nine feet of blood vessel, six hundred pain sensors, nine thousand nerve endings, thirty six heat sensors and seventy five pressure points.

It is important to know that complex carbohydrates (i.e. multi grain breads-48 GI) have a lower glycemic index than simple carbohydrates (i.e. watermelon-72 GI) that generally have a higher glycemic index.

Complex		Simple
0	50	100

H

Halitosis (bad breath) can be caused by the quality of your diet.

Be very careful taking **herbs**. You should consult your doctor for any possible interactions with prescription medications. Children under the age of two (2) should not be given herbal medication.

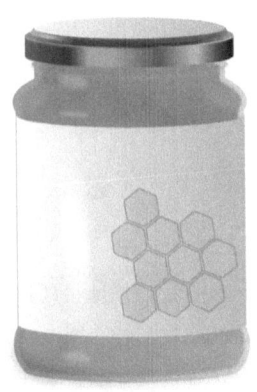

All of the blood in our body passes four hundred times through each kidney per day.

Hydrogenated, partially, fully or "Trans Fats" are highly toxic. Hydrogenated means that hydrogen has been forced into fats and oil, chemically altering the fat so that the body can not use it and it therefore reacts negatively to it.

Honey is a sweet and viscous fluid product produced by honey bees from the nectar of flowers. Honey does not contain any harmful chemicals and is entirely utilized by the digestive tract.

It is recommended to _**not**_ give honey to anyone one year of age or under.

I

Iodine is critical for a properly functioning thyroid.

J

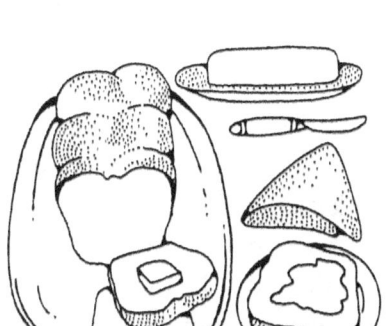

Juices are loaded with sugar so be sure to read labels. Remember a normal serving of orange juice is equivalent to three to five oranges.

K

K= the atomic symbol for potassium which is an important mineral.

L

The **liver** acts as a body detoxifier. It does this by breaking down toxins before they are excreted. The liver plays many roles and is responsible for: converting fat to energy, storing fat soluble vitamins such as A, D, E & K, converting beta carotene to Vitamin A, secreting bile, regulating thyroid function by converting thyroxin into a more usable and active form, and stimulating the intestine by promoting peristalsis, which helps prevent constipation.

M

Don't drink your **milk**. Processing is the problem. During pasteurization, dozens of valuable enzymes are destroyed including lactase for the assimilation of lactose, galactase for the assimilation of galactose, and phosphatase for the assimilation of calcium. Without these enzymes, it makes milk very difficult to digest. All milks apply; non-fat dried milk, and skim milk as well. Cow's milk is rich in phosphorous which can combine with calcium and can prevent you from absorbing the calcium in milk.

Milk is the number one food allergenic in this country. No one needs milk after the age of two. No other mammal on earth continues to drink milk after weaning.

Do not use any form of **margarine**. Margarine was originally manufactured to fatten turkeys. When it killed the turkeys, those involved with the research wanted a monetary return, so they put their heads together to figure out what to do with this product and how to get their money back.

It was a white substance with no food appeal so they added yellow coloring and sold it to people in place of butter. In fact, if you set a tub of margarine outside in a shaded area, no flies will come around it, it will not rot, it will not smell and nothing will grow on it. Why? Because margarine is one molecule away from plastic.

MSG, Monosodium glutamate, was at one time made from seaweed, but now it is made from starch, corn sugar, or molasses from sugar cane or sugar beets. MSG is the sodium salt of glutamate and is simply glutamate, water, and sodium. I recommend the following individuals should avoid MSG; Babies, Children (especially if they have been diagnosed with ADD or ADHD) and pregnant women. Individuals should also avoid MSG if you have been diagnosed with any of the following: Depression, Hypoglycemia, Congestive Heart Failure, Nervous System Disorders, pre-existing Vascular Disease, Renal (kidney) disorders or allergies to MSG. It also adds unnecessary sodium to the diet.

The **microwave** was invented after a researcher walked by a radar tube and a chocolate bar melted in his pocket. Microwaving breaks down the

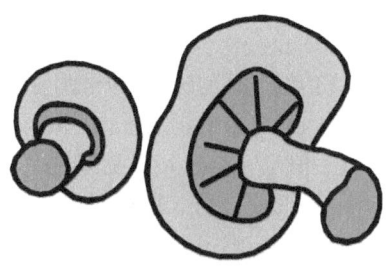

Human Body Trivia:

Your body has about six quarts of blood that circulates through the body three times every minute.

15

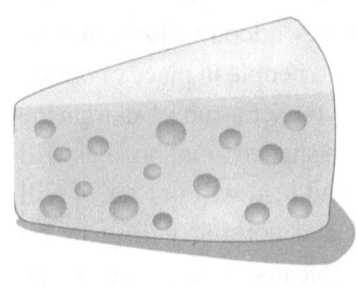

molecular structure of food allowing it to become toxic and leaving it unable for the body to digest.

Mold on cheese can be cut off if it is a small amount. Cut off at least one inch around and below the mold spot (keep the knife out of the mold itself so it will not cross-contaminate other parts of the cheese). Molds that are not part of the manufacturing process can be dangerous. Cheese made with mold are Roquefort, Blue, Gorgonzola, Stilton, Brie and Camembert.

N

The new findings on **neuro toxins** in our food system is important-i. e. cling wraps contain phylates and should not be used near or on food.

Nightshades are tomatoes, potatoes, eggplant and peppers and are so named because they grow in the shade of night. Nightshades contain an alkaloid called solanine, which seems to have a negative effect on calcium in the system.

Nutrition is the study of how food affects our system.

O

Eating **onions** reduces fat droplets in the blood and also tends to dilate blood vessels.

Oils that are recommended are olive oil, extra virgin olive oil (which is never to be heated-just applied to salads) and monounsaturated oil. (Note: Canola oil, although monounsaturated, is a highly refined, genetically-engineered oil with none of the benefits of olive oil).

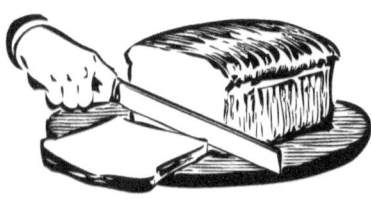

P

Human Body Trivia:

Some causes of stress can be confronted and conquered. Others can be avoided. The best advice: if you can't fight or flee—flow!

Protein is important to the body but remember that your dose is your poison. Too much protein, primarily red meat, can cause the system to be acidic and can slow down the detoxifying of the body.

There are two basic forms of **pasta**-macaroni and noodles. Macaroni products are made from semolina and water. Noodles are made from Durum flour (a more finely ground form of semolina), water, and, by Federal regulation, egg solids. Both are acceptable, especially if made from whole wheat.

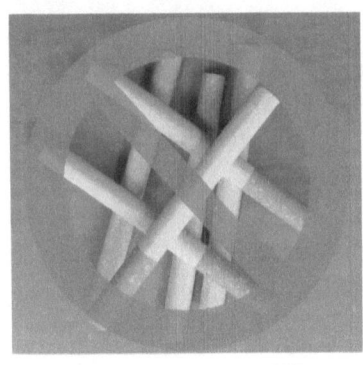

Q

Quit **smoking!** Tobacco leaves are "plumped" by soaking them in Freon (i.e. car refrigerant) and ammonia before freeze drying. Even the paper from a manufactured cigarette contains chemicals, including titanium oxide, which speeds up burning and may contribute to the particular ferocity of fires triggered by burning cigarettes.

Fact:

Diet and physical exercise are key to weight control.

R

Rotate your diet. Any food, if eaten repetitively, has the potential to cause sensitivities in allergy-prone individuals. A diversified rotation of foods will give you the best nutrition possible with the least chance of provoking intolerances and allergies.

Wisdom:

"Our habits will determine the quality of your life."
Anonymous

Learn to **relax**. Meditation and relaxation decreases oxygen consumption, heart rate, respiratory rate and blood pressure. Relaxation helps keep the stress hormone, cortisol, in balance.

S

Eliminate refined **sugars** from the diet. Sugar that quickly enters the blood stream, like processed and

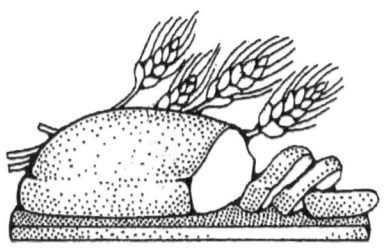

refined sugars, suppress the functioning of the immune system. Sugar feeds bacteria and yeast in the system encouraging disease and oxidation by acidifying the body.

Sugar consumption increases calcium loss.

It is recommended by the National High Blood Pressure Education Program (2002 report) that Americans should consume no more than 2400 mg. of sodium-the equivalent of one teaspoon daily.

Know the other names for sugar when reading labels: dextrose, fructose, maltose, sorghum syrup, corn sweetener, glucose, corn syrup, fruit juice concentrate, honey syrup, high fructose corn syrup, lactose, molasses and brown sugar. Unfortunately the list continues to grow.

Eliminate **stress**. Stress can actually kill, albeit slowly. A study conducted at Ohio State University in 2002, found that even mild stress can increase the risk of cardiovascular disease by leading to above normal levels of homocysteine, an amino acid that damages arterial walls.

Sleep is very important to a healthy system. It is necessary to sleep during

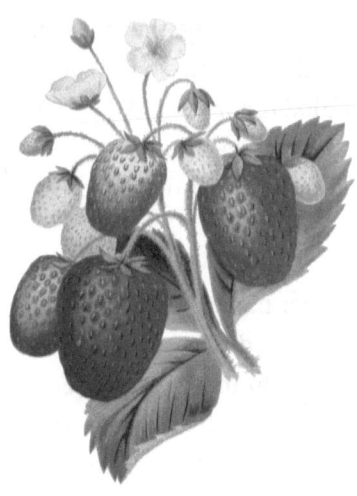

the fourth sleep stage that is generally between 3:00 am and 5:30 am, because this is the time the body does its rebuilding from the day. Waking up during this time consistently, could be attributed to poor nutrition.

Stevia, a sugar substitute, is an herb in the chrysanthemum family that grows wild as a small shrub in parts of Paraquay and Brazil. The glycosides in its leaves account for its incredible sweetness. Stevia is 200-300 times sweeter than table sugar without the negative effects and is now being recommended as the safest form of artificial sweetener.

Splenda, also a sugar substitute, is made of sucralose which was approved in 1998 by the FDA. Unlike other artificial sweeteners, sucralose is made from cane sugar and is 600 times sweeter than sugar itself. Also unlike other sweeteners, it passes through the gastrointestinal tract and the molecules are not absorbed in the body. Anyone allergic to cane sugar will react in the same manner to Splenda.

Serving size is important. Here is a helpful reminder. A deck of cards is a 3 ounce serving of meat, poultry, fish, etc., a regular 60W light bulb is the size of a normal serving of vegetables and a tennis ball represents the size of fruit that is considered a serving.

Take care of your **skin**- it is the largest organ of the body that aids in detoxification along with the liver and the kidneys. Be careful what you rub on your skin as it will be absorbed very quickly by the body. The recommended body and face creams are those that contain vitamins.

SAD is the acronym for Standard American Diet.

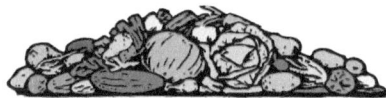

T

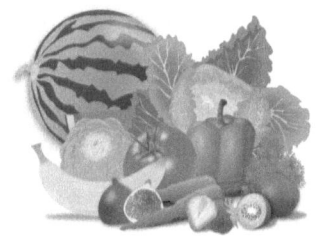

Your **tongue** accurately reflects the state of your digestive system, and all the organs that are associated with blood, nutrient assimilation, and excretion. The tip of the tongue reflects the rectum and descending colon, the peripheral area reflects the large intestine, the middle region corresponds to the small intestine, the back edge region relates to the liver, gallbladder, duodenum, and pancreas,the near back region corresponds to the stomach, the back region (the root of the tongue) reflects the esophagus and the underside of the tongue reflects the quality of blood and lymph circulation in each corresponding area.

<u>Human Body Trivia:</u>

The life span of a taste bud is ten days.

.

The structural characteristics can also reflect the health of the body. A wide tongue indicates an overall balanced physical and psychological disposition. A narrow tongue reflects a lack of physical adaptability with pronounced strengths and weaknesses. A very wide tongue reflects a generally loose and expanded physical condition.

Toxins are potentially harmful substances that occur naturally in twenty percent of foods. Other natural toxins can be produced when food is damaged, or when molds or fungi grow on food. Dried red kidney beans contain natural toxins called lectins, which can cause stomach irritation. These toxins are destroyed if the beans are soaked for at least 12 hours and then boiled vigorously for at least 10 minutes in fresh water. Tinned beans have already undergone this process, although eating out of tins is not recommended. All potatoes contain natural toxins called glycoalkaloids, usually at low levels. Higher levels can be found in green parts of potatoes, sprouted potatoes and potatoes stored in light. It is recommended not to eat potatoes that taste bitter or have a green color on the peel.

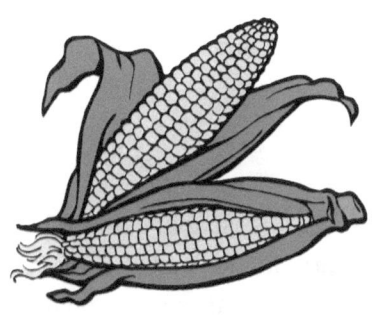

Human Body Trivia:

At birth everyone is color blind.

Moldy or damaged apples may contain a **toxin** called patulin, particularly around the bruised or damaged part of the fruit. It is recommended not to eat this apple or use them to make any type of sauces. Apple seeds contain a naturally occurring substance called amygdalin, therefore it is recommended discarding seeds when juicing apples. Mussels, scallops and oysters are more likely to contain toxins formed by algae in the sea. The greatest risk period of these contaminates is April through September. Molds, known as mycotoxins, can grow on most foods if the conditions are favorable. Even if you remove the mold, it is recommended to throw moldy food away (except previously named cheeses). Toxins are harmful when consumed in larger quantities over a period of time. Following the guidelines listed is the best recommendation for avoiding toxins in foods; Eat a variety of foods (rotate your food), discard foods after the "USE BY" date, and store food properly. Do not assume that natural means safe. Prepare and cook foods properly, discard damaged, discolored foods, and discard foods that smell or have an unusually bitter taste.

U

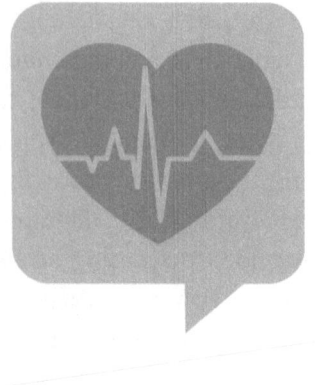

Understanding the role nutrition plays in our health is critical. The American Cancer Society and the National Cancer Institute have both stated that two out of three cancers, diagnosed in 2005, could have been prevented by diet and nutrition alone.

V

Vitamins are essential nutrients and necessary for normal metabolic functions. Vitamins are required daily since the body is unable to store reserves and may make solutions only in water (water-soluble) or in fatty liquids (fat-soluble). Here is a list of water and fat-soluble vitamins. *(For a complete list of vitamins and minerals and how they benefit the body, see page 30.)*

Water Soluble Vitamins (They require water to be absorbed)	Fat Soluble Vitamins (They require fat to be absorbed)
B 7 (Biotin)	Vitamin A
B 12 (Cyanocobalamin)	Vitamin D
B 9 (Folic acid)	Vitamin E
B 3 (Niacin)	Vitamin K
B 5 (Pantothenic Acid)	
B 6 (Pyridoxine)	
B 2 (Riboflavin)	
B 1 (Thiamine)	
Vitamin C	

W

Water-Water-Water.

A rule of thumb on how much water to drink daily- one-half your body weight in ounces of water daily. (i.e. If you weigh one-hundred and twenty pounds, you should drink sixty ounces of water daily). Most daytime fatigue is caused by a lack of water because seventy-five percent of the time-we mistake thirst for hunger.

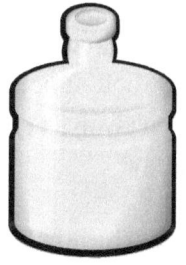

While **water** is important to re-hydrate your system, it is best to limit water (or other liquids) while eating meals. Drinking to much water or other liquids during meal time, dilutes and flushes the food too quickly rather than allowing it to be digested and absorbed properly.

Whole foods are unprocessed foods that have undergone very little processing and have been grown or produced without the use of synthetic pesticides or fertilizers. Synthetic is a process made artificially by synthesis, especially so as to resemble a natural product. Synthetic means that the source is not living food, but dead chemicals. Multi vitamins that are synthetic can be identified by these terms; acetate,

Human Body Trivia:

People are the only animals to cry tears.

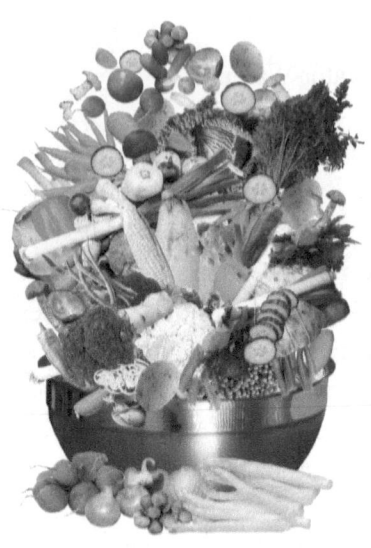

bitartrate, hydrochloride, nitrate, and succinate. Therefore, it is recommended, multi vitamins be whole food supplements.

X Y Z

So, the X Y Z's of The A, B, C's of Nutrition are **X** the following from the diet; alcohol, aluminum, artificial sweeteners, caffeine, canned sodas, MSG, margarine, microwaving, stress and sugar.

Yes to water, whole foods, exercise, relaxation, whole food supplements, rotation of diet, and always remember to eat an apple a day!

Zero in on your own health and listen to your body. Only you can prevent bad health and remember-Prevention saves the body the stress of being sick.

Human Body Trivia:

Every square inch of the human body has an average of thirty two million bacteria on it.

A Rough Guide

*Symptoms that have been related to
foods*

Abdominal Pain   lactose, gluten

Anaphylaxis   wheat, corn, milk, nitrates[6], nightshades
                      (potatoes, tomatoes, eggplant, peppers),
                      cayenne, tobacco, depletion of water from
                      the body

Bed-Wetting   milk, chocolate, citrus juices, tomatoes,
                      pineapple, peaches

Asthma   eggs, nuts, fish, chocolate, gluten, tartrazine
                      (yellow food coloring), benzoates[2], sulphites[7]

Canker Sores   milk, cheese, wheat, tomatoes, vinegar,
                      lemon, pineapple, mustard, gluten

Colds (frequent)   dairy products, sugar, wheat, eggs

Crohn's Disease   gluten, lactose, soy, eggs, milk, tomatoes,
                      nuts

Dermatitis   gluten, milk, eggs

Ear Infections   milk products (Breastfeeding decreases the
                      incidence of infections for the newborn)

Eczema   eggs, milk, wheat, gluten, citrus fruits,
                      tomatoes

Edema	wheat, milk, eggs, corn, coffee, tea, alcohol, yeast, citrus fruits, sugar, tomatoes
Epilepsy	gluten, milk, peanuts, aspartame[1], salicylates
Gallbladder Problems	eggs, pork, onion, poultry, milk, coffee, citrus fruits, corn, beans, nuts
Gastrointestinal	milk, lactose, gluten, sucrose, eggs, nuts, seafood, soy
Gout	purines (meat products, liver, organ meats, sausage, processed meats, anchovies, crab, shrimp), milk, eggs, and a variety of beans.
Hives	gluten, milk, eggs, peanuts, fish, benzoates[2], tartrazine (yellow food coloring[8]), monosodium glutamate[5], sulphites[7]
Hyperactivity	sucrose (sugar), milk, salicylates, BHT[4], BHA[3], artificial colors or flavors[8]
Irregular Heartbeat	milk, eggs
Irritable Bowel	lactose, milk, gluten, wheat, corn, tea, citrus fruit, chicken, eggs, benzoates[2], nitrates[6]
Migraines	cheese, tomatoes, chocolate, coffee, tea, milk, eggs, oranges, wheat, red wine, aspartame[1], tartrazine, tyramines, benzoates[2], nitrates[6], nitrites[6]
Multiple Sclerosis	milk, coffee, chocolate, colas
Psoriasis	gluten

Tinnitus   salicylates

Ulcerative Colon   lactose, milk, gluten

Vasculitis   wine, vinegar

1	Aspartame	artificial chemical sweetener
2	Benzoates	preservatives used in saccharin
3	BHA *(Butylated Hydroxyanisole)*	chemicals that prevents fats, oils and fat
4	BHT *(Butylated Hydroxytoluene)*	containing foods from becoming rancid
5	Monosodium Glutamate *(MSG)*	flavor enhancer used in processed, packaged and fast foods
6	Nitrates / Nitrites	used as preservatives in cured meats to prevent spoilage
7	Sulfites	preserves, dried fruits, shrimp, frozen potatoes
8	Food Colors	used in candy, carbonated drinks, enhances the skin coloring of oranges

Vitamins/Minerals and What They Do

Vitamins

Vitamin A, Antioxidant, and Beta-Carotene
Fat-Soluble

Vitamin A is essential in the formation of visual purple, a pigment found in the retina of the eye that is needed for vision at night. Vitamin A is needed for the health of the outer skin (dermis) and for the body's inner lining. It aids in normal cell reproduction. Approximately 90% of the body's Vitamin A is stored in the liver with small deposits in the fatty tissues, lungs, kidneys, and retinas. Under stressful conditions the body uses this reserve supply if it does not receive enough dietary supplementation. The liver also converts beta carotene to Vitamin A. Carotene is nontoxic, and along with other carotenoids is an antioxidant that offers more protection against cancer than Vitamin A alone.

Excellent Food Sources: beef liver, sweet potatoes, pumpkin, carrots, cantaloupe, winter squash, broccoli, and apricots.

B Complex
Water Soluble

Foods that are especially rich in one of the B Complex vitamins will also contain several other members of the complex as their functions in the body are also closely interrelated.

They are NOT stored in the body in any great quantity and need to be supplied by the diet. The need for the complex increases during chronic illnesses, stress, and when alcohol, tobacco and drugs are used. Taking

B complex, which includes the whole B vitamin family, will lessen the chance of an imbalance or deficiency of a single B vitamin.

Thiamine (Vitamin B1)
Water Soluble

Mental efficiency, health and a feeling of well being are dependent on thiamine. Thiamine is required for the nerve cells to function properly. It is essential for the formation of ATP (adenosine triphosphate), the energy fuel that the body runs on, in every cell. Another vital role of B 1 is its importance in normal metabolism which is the rate at which calories are burned by the body to function normally.

Excellent Food Sources: sunflower seeds, pecans, pork, peanuts, green peas, bran flakes, and ham.

Riboflavin (Vitamin B2)
Water Soluble

Riboflavin is a constituent of enzymes involved in cell respiration. Riboflavin contributes to the growth and repair of the cell tissue throughout the body, especially the skin, mucous membranes, and eyes. The vitamin converts carbohydrates to ATP during its metabolism of proteins, carbohydrates and fats.

Excellent Food Sources: brewer's yeast, liver, heart, and kidney meats, milk, sardines, and cheese.

Niacin (Vitamin B3)
Water Soluble

Niacin is a coenzyme involved in the metabolism of proteins, fats, and carbohydrates. Besides its presence in food, the vitamin is manufactured in the body from the essential amino acid tryptophan. It is important for blood circulation and reducing cholesterol levels in the blood.

Excellent Food Sources: roasted peanuts, chicken, beef liver, turkey, tuna, salmon, sunflower seeds, and raw oysters.

Pyridoxine (Vitamin B6)
Water Soluble

Pyridoxine is extremely important in the development of the nervous system. It helps process amino acids and is involved in the production of serotonin, melatonin, and dopamine. The vitamin has been used to reduce morning sickness during pregnancy. It is also beneficial for PMS, nerve compression injuries, and carpal tunnel syndrome. Because of its role in fat metabolism, a deficiency can increase the amount of fatty build up in the arteries. A lack of the vitamin can also be associated with depression.

Excellent Food Sources: brewer's yeast, toasted wheat germ, sunflower seeds, beef liver, and soybeans.

Cyanocobalamin (Vitamin B12)
Water Soluble

Absorption of B12 depends on the presence in the stomach of the intrinsic factor, a mucoprotein enzyme. Autoimmune reactions in the body may bind the intrinsic factor to prevent B12 absorption or prevent cellular ability to produce the enzyme. It also helps iron function better in the body. B 12 is necessary for the functioning of all body cells, especially those of the bone marrow, nervous system, and gastrointestinal tract.

Excellent Food Sources: liver, raw clams, raw oysters, and herring.

Folic Acid (Vitamin B9)
Water Soluble

Folic acid is involved in the duplication of chromosomes during cell reproduction, a process that is accelerated during pregnancy when new tissue is being formed. The vitamin is important in preventing birth abnormalities such as neural tube defects, which involves poor brain and spinal cord development. It can help in preventing cleft palate. Folic acid regulates blood homocysteine levels, an amino acid associated with the increased risk of heart disease, strokes, osteoporosis, and Alzheimer's. It is necessary for the production of the mood related substance SAMe.

Excellent Food Sources: wheat germ, brewer's yeast, broccoli, liver, and spinach.

Pantothenic Acid (Vitamin B5)
Water Soluble

There is a close correlation between pantothenic acid tissue levels and functioning of the adrenal glands which are important in responding to stress. It is involved in cholesterol and hormone synthesis. Fifty percent of pantothenic acid is lost in the milling of grains and thirty seven percent during the cooking process of meat.

Excellent Food Sources: yeast, egg yolks, beef liver, wheat bran, wheat germ, and sunflower seeds.

Biotin (Vitamin B7)
Water Soluble

Biotin acts as a coenzyme in the metabolism of fats, carbohydrates, and protein. Prolonged use of antibiotics and anti-seizure medicines interfere with its production. The vitamin strengthens brittle nails and lowers blood glucose levels preventing diabetic neuropathy. Deficiency symptoms include fatigue, lack of appetite, dermatitis, hair loss, anemia, nausea, and depression.

Excellent Food Sources: liver, egg yolks, nuts, cauliflower, legumes, and mushrooms.

Choline and Inositol

These vitamins are constituents of lecithin and are primarily associated with the use of fats and cholesterol in the body and for cell membrane integrity. Choline is a component of acetylcholine, a neurotransmitter in the brain, and has been helpful in treating neurological and psychological disorders. Inositol is also involved in nerve transmission. Diabetics excrete inositol at a rate greater than normal.

Excellent Food Sources: egg yolks, beef liver, whole grains, wheat germ and most meats.

Vitamin C, Antioxidant
Water Soluble

Vitamin C is necessary for the formation of collagen, the connective tissue in skin, ligaments, and bones, and is important for the healing of wounds. The vitamin aids in forming red blood cells and preventing hemorrhaging and bleeding gums. It maintains the activity of white blood cells which act as bacteria fighters, but too high amounts of C reverse that effect and white bloods cells actually become less active.

Vitamin C has shown protective effects against heavy metal exposure, pesticides, and food additives such as nitrates, which have been associated with cancer. Birth control pills and aspirin deplete the tissue of Vitamin C. It protects against free radicals as described earlier.

Vitamin D
Fat Soluble

Vitamin D is necessary for the absorption of calcium from the intestinal tract reducing its urinary excretion, and for the assimilation of phosphorous which is required in bone formation. When skin is exposed to ultraviolet radiation, vitamin D is formed from a cholesterol derivative and absorbed into the circulatory system. The more pigment there is in the skin, less of the vitamin is produced. Vitamin D is involved in cell reproduction, blood cell formation, and enhances it the immune system.

Vitamin E, Antioxidant
Fat Soluble

Vitamin E plays an essential role in cellular respiration of all muscles. This makes it possible for muscles and their nerves to function with less oxygen, thereby increasing endurance and stamina. Vitamin E is mainly found in the oily portions of foods like whole grains and seeds. High doses interfere with iron metabolism. It protects against free radicals.

Vitamin K
Fat Soluble

Vitamin K is necessary for the formation of prothtrombin, a chemical required in blood clotting. Besides dietary sources, it is manufactured in the intestinal tract by certain bacteria. Vitamin K can interfere with the actions of some blood thinners.

Minerals

Calcium

Calcium is the most abundant mineral in the body. 98% is found in the bones, 1% in the teeth, and 1% in other tissues. Calcium helps regulate nerve transmission along with magnesium, and is important in cardiovascular health. If muscles do not have enough calcium, they cannot contract. The converse is true if contracted-they cannot relax, which results in cramping. The mineral is good for relaxation and improves the quality of sleep. During the hormonal shift of menopause, the dominance of the parathyroid hormone causes calcium to be removed from bone resulting in osteoporosis. High intake of calcium interferes with the absorption of other minerals including iron, zinc, and manganese, disrupts the functioning of the nervous and muscular systems, and may prevent blood coagulation.

Chromium

A trace element, chromium is essential in producing a substance called glucose tolerance factor (GTF) which is important in the utilization of insulin, a hormone that stabilizes blood sugar levels. The mineral is also involved in the synthesis of fatty acids and cholesterol. Eating refined sugar can cause depletion of body chromium, as sugar lacks sufficient amounts of the mineral for its own digestion.

Copper

Copper assists in the formation of hemoglobin and red blood cells by facilitating the absorption of iron and may protect against arteriosclerosis. Iron metabolism depends on copper. Zinc and copper have similar elemental properties and have a balancing effect on each other. High levels of copper may aggravate PMS. Excess copper can cause mental and emotional problems and can be prominent in schizophrenia. Excess copper may be getting into the diet from contaminated food and water sources, such as copper pipes through which drinking water flows.

Iodine

Iodine aids in the development and functioning of the thyroid gland and is an integral part of thyroxine, a principal hormone produced by the thyroid.

Iron

At the center of a hemoglobin molecule is iron and when combined with oxygen, it gives arterial blood its bright red color. Iron is also necessary for the formation of myoglobin, found only in muscle tissue, which supplies oxygen to the muscle cells. Significant amounts of iron can be lost during menstruation and needs are higher for pregnant women. Excess iron can accumulate in the body to toxic levels.

Magnesium

Along with zinc, magnesium lowers serum copper levels and balances histamine levels, a substance that is released during allergic reaction. Magnesium also helps maintain glucose levels.

Potassium and Sodium

Potassium and sodium exist in important ratios with potassium concentrated inside the cells and sodium remaining outside. They regulate water balance in the body and their equilibrium enables them to stimulate nerve impulses for the heart and other muscle contractions. Depletion of either element depresses cell response. The typical American diet of processed and convenience foods do not contain sufficient amounts of potassium creating an imbalance between the two minerals. Diuretics can cause an excessive urinary loss of potassium. An excess of sodium is related to high blood pressure and fluid retention which inhibit the role of the heart and kidneys.

Selenium, Antioxidant

Selenium is a natural antioxidant and appears to preserve the elasticity of tissues by delaying oxidation of polyunsaturated fatty acids. It supports the immune system, protects against cancer, is a factor in infertility, and is necessary for the production of prostaglandin, a substance that affects blood pressure.

Selenium content of foods is dependant on the soil and according to the most recent research by the USDA, the soil in the United States is almost totally depleted of selenium.

Zinc

Zinc is a constituent of at least 25 enzymes involved in digestion and metabolism. It is a component of insulin and essential in the synthesis of nucleic acids which control the formation of different proteins in the cell. The mineral speeds the healing of wounds and bone fractures, keeps the skin healthy, and is involved in the formation of keratin, a substance in hair and nails. Zinc also supports the immune system and protects against free radicals.

Mediterranean Type Diet Recommendations

HOW TO EAT

1) Eat every two hours. This eliminates stress formation in the body maintaining normal blood sugar levels between meals.

2) Do not eat carbohydrates alone; always add protein to your meals and snacks. It is especially important not to eat a breakfast composed of carbohydrates solely.

3) Avoid stimulants-caffeine, sugar, alcohol, etc. Stimulants work by provoking the stress handling glands into releasing epinephrine and cortisol to raise blood sugar and release energy or ATP which is vital to maintain proper metabolic reactions which will therefore slow down metabolism and may lead to weight gain.

4) Avoid dead, devitalized and junk food. These foods cannot re-build a healthy body. They are also anti-nutrients. They steal any remaining nutrient stores from your body and may contain MSG which should also be avoided.

5) Avoid trans-fats and rancid fats. Cell membranes, nerve tissue, and steroid hormones (vitality hormones) all require healthy fats. Unhealthy fats interfere with bodily functions and structures.

6) Eat real, whole, fresh food. Minimize fruit and fruit juices. Most people will do well on a Mediterranean-type diet, combining some carbohydrates, protein, and fat at each meal.

7) Salt your food with sea salt. Stress handling glands need salt for normal function. Low salt diets can contribute to adrenal fatigue.

8) Drink plenty of water (preferably filtered, or a reliable source of spring water, NOT tap water which may contain an abundance of heavy metals from water pipes).

WHAT TO EAT

1) Eat foods rich in Omega 3 fatty acids such as fatty coldwater (not farm grown) fish, including salmon, tuna, herring and mackerel. Eat walnuts, flaxseeds and green leafy vegetables.
2) Use monounsaturated oils, especially olive oil (extra virgin olive can be used but it is not designed to be heated) as your primary oil/ fat source.
3) Eat seven or more servings of fresh vegetables and fruits daily. Fresh or frozen are preferred over canned. Vegetables can be slightly cooked, steamed or eaten raw.
4) Eat natural sources of good protein (not man made deli meats), preferably organic or free range meats.
5) Eat more protein from vegetables: including peas, beans lentils, and nuts.
6) Eat only organic whole grains. No refined carbohydrates (i.e. white flour, white rice, white pasta, white sugar).
7) The best breads are found in the frozen section of the store. Look for organic sprouted grain breads (sprouted grains have a higher protein and lower carbohydrate content than regular flour). These must be kept refrigerated.
8) Minimize oils that are high in Omega 6 fatty acids, including corn, safflower, sunflower, soybean, and cottonseed oils.
9) Reduce or eliminate intake of trans-fatty acids (all hydrogenated oils), which are prevalent in margarine, vegetable shortening, and almost all commercially prepared packaged foods.
10) Make complex carbohydrates (such as breads, pasta, and grains) your smallest food group.

Food Combining Groups

High-Starch	_Non-Starch_	_High-Protein_	_Fruits_
grains	asparagus	beans	apricot
pastas	broccoli	legumes	banana
rice	Brussel sprouts	fish	berries
corn	cabbage	poultry	cherry
potato (all)	cauliflower	wild game	date
turnip	celery, chives	meat (all)	lemon
squash	cucumber	seafood	grapefruit
parsnip	kale, kohlrabi	seeds	mango
beet	leeks	nuts	melons (all)
carrots	leafy greens	dairy products	nectarine
eggplant	onions		pineapple
avocado	peppers (all)		papaya
	parsley, radishes		peach
	zucchini		pear
	watercress		plum
	green beans		tomato
	artichokes		apply
	sea vegetables		fig
	dandelion greens		orange
	endive, okra		
	swiss chard		

DISCLAIMER:

The information contained in this book is provided for informational and educational purposes only, and is not intended to convey medical advice or to substitute for advice from your own physician. This information is not intended to diagnose, treat, cure or prevent any disease or condition. The information presented herein is not intended to be a substitute for medical counseling. Always consult a doctor or nutritional consultant before making any dietary changes or taking any nutritional supplement(s).

References

Colbert, Don, M.D. *What You Don't Know May Be Killing You.* 2004. Siloam, A Strang Company, Wheaton, IL, 60189

Todd, Gary Price, M.D. *Nutrition, Health & Disease,* 1985. Whitford Press, a division of Schiffer Publishing, Ltd., Atglen, PE, 19310.

Murray, Michael T., N.D. *Natural Alternatives To Over-The Counter And Prescription Drugs.* 1999. Quill. New York.

Batmanghelidj, F.M.D., *You're Not Sick, You're Thirsty.* 2003. Warner Books. New York.

Simopoulos, Artemis P., M.D., and Jo Robinson, *The Omega Diet: The Lifesaving Nutritional Program Based on the Diet of the Island of Crete.* 1999. Harper Collins Publishers, Inc.

Chi, Tsu-Tsair, Ph. D., *Dr. Chi's Method of Fingernail and Tongue Analysis.* 2002.

Chi Enterprise.

Griffith, H. Winter, M.D., *Revised Edition, Vitamins Herbs, Minerals and Supplements, The Complete Guide.* 1998. DaCapo Press. Cambridge, MA.

www.weightloss.about.com/gi/dynamic/offsite

Lang, Janet R., D.C., *The Cardiovascular Seminar.* 2006. Lang Integrated Health Seminar LLC.

www.medindia.net

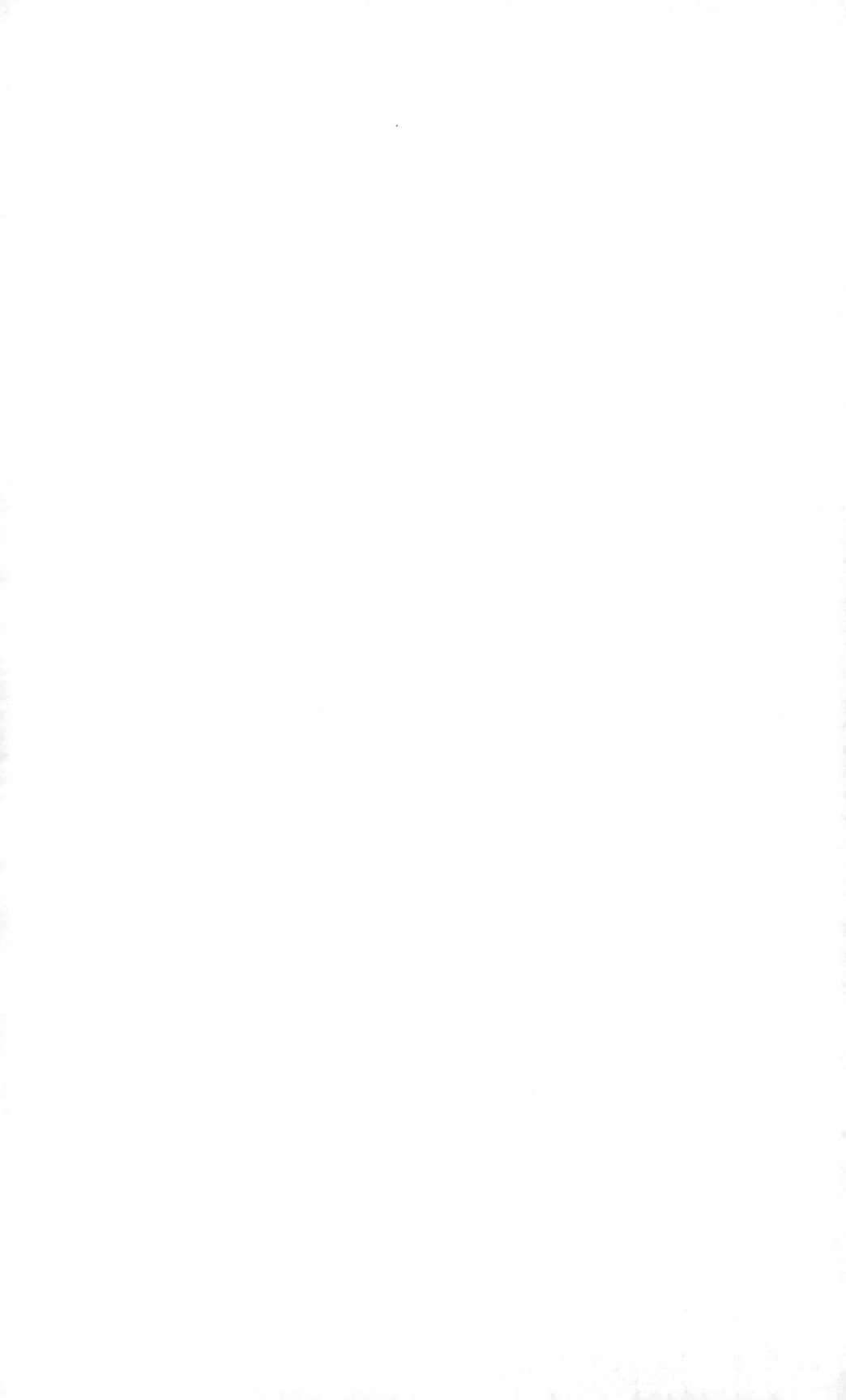